TEN WAYS OF HEALTH

THE HYGIENIC SYSTEM REVISITED

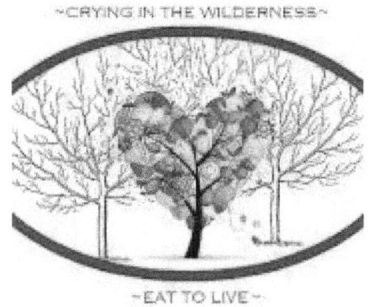

FERRANTE FRAZIER, M.S., C.H.N.P., C.N.H.P.

Many persons bring disease upon themselves by their self-indulgence. They have not lived in accordance with natural law. Others have disregarded the Laws of Health in their habits of eating and drinking, dressing or working. Often some form of vice is the cause of the feebleness of mind or body. Should these persons gain the blessing of health, many of them would continue to pursue the same course of heedless transgression of God's natural and spiritual laws, reasoning that if God heals them in answer to prayer, they are at liberty to continue their unhealthful practices and to indulge perverted appetites without restraints if God were to work a miracle in restoring these persons to health, He would simply be encouraging their unhealthful living habits.

~Ellen White, 1900~

Ellen White knew the true cause of disease and the restoration process. She realized that all our diseases are linked directly to our personal habits and environmental conditions. If the SUPREME BEING would grant forgiveness for breaking the laws that were created by Him, then He would be aiding in the breaking of the law. Why obey a law that can easily be forgiven with a prayer? We might as well break the law and immediately ask for forgiveness. The law then is made of no effect to us. This is the same as making it a law that says that speeding is prohibited, but the penalties can be forgiven with an "I'm sorry." Why should we ever worry about getting caught for speeding if we can get out of every penalty for breaking the law by apologizing?

3

The same is true with medicine, herbs, supplements, therapeutic agencies or treatments and surgery. Our health issues are directly related to our personal habits and environmental conditions. When our habits and environmental conditions violate the laws governing our bodies, dis-ease will be the result of such disobedience. When our habits and environmental conditions do not violate the laws governing the body, vibrant health and longevity will be the result of such obedience. When the medical and herbal doctors provide you with medicine or herbs in which to suppress or palliate your symptoms of dis-ease, he/she is also encouraging the habits and environmental conditions that produced the dis-ease to be continued. This means that the doctor and the patient are unaware of the true nature of dis-ease.

A man notices that, after eating his usual meal that he has been eating for years, his stomach has a bloating and burning sensation in it. He refers to family, friends or advertisements to find the best form of relief from his di-ease. He is told about over-the-counter or herbal remedies to stop the dis-comforts so that he can enjoy his usual meal like he use to. His usual meals are the reason for his dis-comforts but he takes a remedy to palliate or suppress the symptoms. After awhile, he learns that he has an ulcer in the stomach. Little did he know that the palliative measure was as smart as cutting the fire alarm off without putting out the fire. In fact, instead of putting out the fire, more gasoline was poured onto the fire by having the ability to eat more from the suppressive means of the medicine. The burning sensations did not stop, only the pain was silenced. The burning sensation was the mixture in the stomach

4

burning a whole in it. When the man first felt the pain, he could not eat; but when he suppresses the pain, he was able to resume his bad habit of eating. Remedies encouraged his bad eating.

Pain is our guardian angel. Without it we would get into a lot of situations that would destroy us. If we were to approach heat, we would feel the pain of it as we get closer and closer to it. If the pain was not felt, we would be in the fire before we could do something about it. Diabetics are warned to check themselves often to make sure that they haven't bruised themselves. These people have lost the ability to feel sensation in the nerves. This means that they cannot feel pain like regular people. In fact, they can step on a nail and not be aware that they did unless they check often. This must mean that pain prevents damage and lets us know when we have been damage. Why should we silence our alarm without finding the cause, and then removing it, of the thing that set off the alarm?

I dedicate this book to all those people who wish to live healthy long lives by removing the cause of dis-ease.

INTRODUCTION

Since my teenage years, I have searched every means by which to lose the morbid weight I had accumulated. I tried all of the prevailing diets, and I had my share of "detoxes" that only forced my bowels to void its contents. I went from eating the standard American diet to eating the ideal diet design to provide the body with the greatest health attainable. I went from no exercise to routinely exercising.

I had managed to reach an all time high scale reading of three hundred and fifty-three pounds. This was the most miserably time of my life, because my energy level was very low and my body was very unattractive. Even going in stores to find clothes that fit me was humiliating, because I could never find anything big enough that would fit me that look decent to wear. Most stores did not carry the plus sizes; and if they did, they were not appealing and few in pieces. This meant that all the big guys would be wearing pretty much the same outfit. Not to forget to mention the price of the plus-sized clothing, but they were usually double or triple the price of regular clothes. The morbid weight kept me humiliated; and when not humiliated, it kept me broke. At times, it kept me broke and humiliated.

Weight was just one of the many problems that I suffered from in the past. My health was deteriorating at a rapid rate with no cause identified. At the age of eighteen when I should have been enjoying the health of my youth, I was already dealing with type 2 diabetes(adult onset.) This was

6

before I was considered an adult. I was told that I had high blood pressure. I was diagnosed with asthma and I would frequently get nose bleeds.

By the time I reached the age of thirty, I started having fatigue and failure in the sex organs; however, there were stimulants that kept them working even when they were begging to be left alone to rest. This could explain the reason for the vital exhaustion in the whole body. Shortly after the chronic fatigue started, I started feeling pins and needle-like sensations in both of my legs. The sensations would increase in severity as the evening progressed, and it would be unbearable at night. Seems like the only time I was not in pain was when I was able to fall asleep and when I got up in the mornings. The health 'experts' were telling me that I was suffering with neuropathy. However, it was in my hands as well as the feet. The sensations ran at the same time on the left as it did on the right. When one of the hands felt numb and tingly, so did the other one feel numb and tingly; and the same goes for both of the feet. Looking back at the suffering, I am inclined to believe that it was the body drawing its energy from less vital areas to areas of more importance since I was reaching chronic fatigue. The energy needed for functioning power is termed nervous or vital energy in Hygiene. I will explain nerve energy in more details latter in this reading.

I followed the medical mentality at the first onset of my health issues. I inhaled the asthma inhalers and took the breathing treatments like a good disciple. I regularly swallowed the medicines for the high blood pressure, high blood sugar and pain. Even when those didn't remove the

7

cause of dis-ease, but instead made it worse, I resulted to the remedies and concoctions of the alternative 'natural' health profession. Of the herbal remedies and modalities, I followed and ingested them as a faithful student of alternative care. I studied the use of many of the remedies and 'natural' treatments. Although I was obedient to the medical and herbal mentality, they both turned out to be a complete failure. None of those mentalities addressed the cause of my suffering. They only addressed the symptoms and the application by which to suppress and deal with the suffering while allowing me to continue the lifestyle that I was living that produced the suffering. Not only did I pay dearly financially, but I squandered away my energy and health by suppressing my illnesses while the cause of the illnesses was still present.

With so many health education concepts in my brain, it was amazing how my situation got worse. When all forms of attempts to remove my suffering failed, I came across a system of care like no other. It was only after I tried everything did I learn about the "DO NOTHING" system. The only things that were required in the "DO NOTHING" system was to find and remove the cause. Once the cause is removed, we should supply the body with the means and influences that is required for health. These means and influences will be presented to you as the ten ways of health. I did not invent these ten ways, but rather learned them during my search for health. They are required for the healthy to have health and for the sick to regain health.

As I write this, I am currently healthy and full of vitality. All of the health issues that I describe earlier are long forgotten in the ancient past. In other words, I am no longer a member of the suffering class that is searching for a savior to their woes. My weight has reached and maintained itself at an ideal mark of around 185 pounds. I now have trouble finding small clothes in which to wear, but I contributed that to the clothing companies are making their clothes to fit what our society has become – out of shape obese people. Obesity has become so common that a majority of the clothing manufacturers are answering the cries from the consumers to 'cover up' our huge bodies. The clothes in the stores are now huge in the waist but short in the length of them. They are getting wider and growing less. This means that the regular American of today is growing out instead of growing up.

This system of care of which I am sharing with you has worked with all those who learn and apply it to their lives. Just reading this book without applying the ways spoke of, herein, will not bring about the success that it has the ability to bring to those who apply them in good faith. It reminds me of a cartoon of my youth that would always say, "Knowing is half the battle." The name of the cartoon was *G.I. JOE*. To know is just half of what you have to do to bring about a change. Application is the other half of the battle if we wish to get results from what has been learned from these pages.

The knowledge of health is within these pages. Don't just be a reader of these words, but be a doer also. There are ten ways or ingredients for health. Each way or ingredient must be used to bring about the best health possible. To only use a couple and not all may leave you still suffering. Imagine baking a cake that consists of ten ingredients. Now, imagine only using five out of the ten of the ingredients to bake the cake. What do you think will be the outcome of the cake? Certain ingredients cannot be left out at all while others will only destroy the cakes taste, color, etc. This is the same with the ingredients or ways of health. Some are more needed then the others; but without the others, life would not be a great tasting cake. You get the point. Practice all ten of theses simple ways of health and reap the joy of vibrant health and longevity.

As you continue to read this text, you may get the impression that I hate doctors. That would not be true, because I only have fault with the cure mongers and drug dealers that exploit sufferers with their poisons. Their suppression and palliation of minor illnesses causes major ones to develop. This means that their meddling with acute dis-eases cause them to become chronic. The acute dis-ease is the body initiated response to free itself from a toxic environment. Look at the alcoholic who poisons themselves with toxic drinks. After consumption of the poisons, the body develops a crisis to eliminate the poisons. It causes the kidneys to filter more of the toxins out of the blood; it causes sweating to eliminate toxins from the skin; it causes the digestive system to flush it out of the bowels or regurgitate it up through the throat. The alcoholic has headaches, nausea and many other symptoms of dis-ease. This should mean that all acute dis-eases are from poisoning – from within or without. Is their a cure, drug, herb that can sober the drunk man while he continues to drink? NO! I find fault with those doctors that makes the suffering class believe that their dis-eases can be cured while they continue

10

in the habits that produced and caused them. Nothing is to say that I am against those doctors that preform emergency surgery to revive a stopped heart.

I wrote this that you may know the true and only ways of health. Any way that denies fresh air, pure water, adequate sunlight, internal and external cleanliness, rest and relaxation, regular exercise and mobility, normal temperatures, ideal foods designed for the human body, emotional balance with control of the passions and nurturing relationships is not true and should not be trusted. All the ways to health are true according to their agreement to those ten ways of health.

I am not a medical or herbal doctor, and neither do I hold myself out to be a member of the cure mongers. So, if you feel that you have a condition that requires medicine, herbs, supplements, or therapeutic agencies and treatments, you should consult a medical doctor, herbal doctor, or any of the other doctors that are in the curing business. We do not cure anything. We believe that the body cures itself when the cause/causes are removed and the ten ways of health are practiced. We do not believe that there is any substance that can cure the body when sick, for we believe that the substance will only suppress and palliate. If disease is right action, and it is, then it should not be stopped. Only thing that the body requires to regain health is removal of cause and obedience to the ten ways of health.

Dis-ease is right action. Remember when I said that acute dis-eases were a response from the body to eliminate toxins from the internal environment? Well, that is considered right action. When the alcoholic threw up, was that right

11

action or wrong action? Let's see: What would happen if the alcoholic didn't sweat or urinate out the toxins; what if the toxins were allowed to stay in the body? It may cause possible death within minutes. Picture someone ingesting rat poison. The person is rush to the emergency room to have their stomach pumped or given something to stop it from being taken into the blood. The more volatile a poison is, the more violent will the body act in self defense to maintain its integrity. When we sneeze in a dust storm, this should be viewed as right action; because it is freeing the dust from the lungs and bronchial tract. When we sneeze to release toxic mucus that is being eliminated via abnormal routes, why should we think that the sneezing is wrong action? The sneezing is triggered by the presence of something that irritates the lining of the respiratory tract. Should this action be stopped with medicine, herbs or any other substance or treatment? Absolutely not! How will the body free itself from the toxins? The toxins will be stored in the body causing all kinds of havoc. Suppression of acute dis-eases is a co-producer of chronic dis-eases.

PART ONE

UNDERSTANDING OUR SYSTEM

The Hygienic System Revised

As I stated earlier, I am not a medical doctor or an herb man, so nothing in this book will encourage the intake of any medicines or herbs. I will only teach the true cause of dis-ease and the means by which to remove its symptoms from the body provided that the cells of the body hasn't reach a point of no return. Where this system of care fails to restore health back, all others are bound to fail or have already failed.

This book is not for the medical profession who are devoted to their drug and treatment applications with hopes to restore health. No, this book is for those common people who prefer the correct education on the true ways of living to bring about health in all its virtue. The aim of this book is to free the sufferer from praying to the drug pushers for relief from their woes. This book is to stop the butchers from destroying the integrity of a whole body with the scalpel and knife. It starts with you reading, understanding, and applying these ways of health that you avoid sickness. To avoid sickness will run those in the curing business out of business.

The medical profession, with their modern education and propaganda, teaches us that dis-ease must be cured or prevented using medicine or the knife in surgery; so they emphasize antibodies and immunization programs and the dangers of bad violent micro-organisms called germs, bacteria and viruses. Instead of telling us about the right way to live that we prevent disease, they teach wrongly about dis-ease prevention that people may continue their dis-ease producing behavior with a false sense of security. What is the prevention of drunkenness? Is it not to refrain from drinking? Prevention is brought about by abstaining from the thing that will cause it.

The Hygienic system of care is based on the value of cleanliness, sunshine, rest, and other proper living habits that the healthy and sick body needs. The only difficulty in teaching a newcomer the ten ways of health is that they have learned a whole lot of medical falsehoods from all avenues in their lives. In school from kindergarten on to college, we have been taught the medical understanding of "health education," which is no difference then the advertising commercials they teach through the television and radio airwaves.

Most people are brainwashed in the medical falsehoods and are closed to new truth. The only way to get rid of a headache is an aspirin, B.C. powder, Tylenol, etc., etc. to these people. Does the body have aspirin, Aleve, Tylenol, B.C. powder reserve levels in it, and when low, produce headaches that require their intake to stop the headache? Can taking the medicines prevent a headache? How is it that a headache is "cured" with the use of one pill, and then later it requires two, three and then four or more to bring about relief? Is the medicine losing its power? Why doesn't newborns and children required to take these pills to prevent them from ever developing a headache?

We would think that the educated medical profession and other health professions should know these simple

15

truths that you will learn in this book, but many fools pass as wise men solely because they hold a degree in their respected field. This only means that they learn everything that the college they attended thought to be important. The problem starts with the education. They are educated in the wrong direction. The foundation of their studies is not solid. They are looking for dis-ease as being caused from some external entity or it being something to cure. Those whose foundation is built on searching for external causes and external cures will never understand that we build our own dis-ease by our personal habits and environmental conditions; so, they will never look at the habits or environment of the sick, but would rather search for germs and viruses and search for cures outside of the body.

Dis-ease is the result of wrong personal habits or environmental conditions that weaken the vitality of the body. When this vitality becomes low, the organs falter in their job. The elimination organs are usually the first to become fatigue. When they become fatigued, they are unable to eliminate toxins from the blood. The toxins begin to accumulate in the blood poisoning the body from within. The poison starts to irritate the cells they come in contact with. This causes the cells to become inflamed, or what doctors call inflammation. The inflammation is the cause of the discomforts and pain of dis-ease. It also leads to ulceration and then to induration(hardening.) The hardening causes the cells to degenerate and die.

The medical mentality believes that dis-ease is inevitable and is caused by some germ or virus that crawled under our fingernails or came from the shake of a hand. This is

16

opposite to our system of understanding, for we believe that the symptoms of dis-ease can be avoided or reversed if the individual will practice the ten proper lifestyle habits to not produce dis-ease in them. In other words, the medical "expert's" education has not educated them. In fact, it has them on a wild goose chase for the Boogieman, Bigfoot and the Loch Ness Monster.

The experts are not thinking for themselves. They are rather textbook slaves reciting the Latin and Greek terms they have been studying for years. At best, they are good language interpreters; although, truth seems to get lost in their translation.

The average sufferer of today doesn't seem to want to think for themselves either. We have placed all of our trust in doctors, pills, and potions to keep us healthy and return us to health when we become sick. We have been taught to not ask or question the doctor's authority. We are encouraged to take digestive and gastric pills so that we can continue our bad eating. Why aren't we encouraged to eat right to not suffer the digestive problems that wrong eating causes? We are told to be good listeners. However, in this book, we refuse to listen and recite their understanding of dis-ease that requires the ingesting of poisonous drugs and destructive means from the cutting of surgery. We are revealing truth to those who love truth wherever truth lies. After reading this book, you the reader, will know the truth about how to get well and stay well without the medicine or herbal man. A proverb says, "And the truth shall set you free." Once you learn the truth about the cause and nature of dis-ease, you will understand how to avoid and reverse it.

17

This will free you from the captive understanding of the medical mentality.

Be excited that you have found this book; for in doing so, you have stumble upon the true means to real health. All of your searching for health has led you to this system of care. Had the other systems had any worth, your search would have ended long ago. Although, our system was here before the first human existed, for it is a system of growth, development and reproduction. Our system is a true science for health based on the natural laws of life. If one doesn't obey this system, di-ease will become the rule. If one obeys this system, health will become the rule.

Medicine is not and never will be a science. It is merely a manner or method of treating the sick. Physiology, biology, anatomy, etc., are sciences, because their principles can be demonstrated, but these are not medicine. Yes, physicians are required to study these sciences, but medicine is not based on them. They also have to take courses understanding medicine and its application. Medicine has no principle that can be demonstrated. That's why ten people can take the same medicine and it can affect each one differently. This is not true with fresh air, or the other ways of health. The medical modes of treatment are short-lived, which would not be true if they were truly a science. This is why they claim to practice medicine. There is no specific outcome from taking a medicine. This means that it cannot be a true science. Gravity is able to be demonstrated every time, for what goes up must come down. In medicine, they say that an outcome should or might happen. That's

18

why they say let's try you on this pill to see what it does. This is not a science.

Everything about the medical profession is experimental. They inform you that they are practicing medicine. Well, when is the practicing over with? It's time to stop practicing and get in the game of health restoration and stop the suppression and palliation.

As I stated earlier, what good is listening to our experts of today if what they are teaching us is not true or based on sound science? Our system provides you with the true knowledge of the ten ways of health. Don't let this truth interfere with the image of yourself. We should not be too proud to admit we have been wrong in our understanding of health in the past. Another proverbs come to mind, "Unless you become a child(unlearned) again, you cannot inherit the kingdom of God." You cannot hear truth if your ears are blocked or full of untruths. When the ears are unlearned, only then will we be willing to accept the new truths; not new to existence, but new to your attention. We will not continue to seek health from poisonous drugs, as we do not seek warmth from the air conditioner but rather the heater. We will employ the ten natural ways to restore health to our bodies.

Doctors give medicine to suppress or palliate symptoms so that their patient can return and continue their daily routine, without having the dis-comforts that comes from the habits of their daily routine. They don't understand that it is their daily routine that is causing their dis-ease. Imagine the alcoholic who doesn't realize what is keeping him drunk. Imagine him blaming it on some tiny or unseen entity.

19

Suppressing the symptoms without removing the cause, as the medical mentality so often do, leaves them in their dis-ease producing habits.

The medical mentality way of health is the cause of the more chronic issues. As the cause continue, the condition of the sufferer gets worse. The worse the condition becomes, the more the attempt to stop the symptoms with drugs and surgery. Let's look at something as simple as eyeglasses: the patient has a not so strong prescription, but every year or two they will have to go to the eye doctor to get a stronger lens(so much for CORRECTIVE lens, because they correct nothing) due to the worsening of their sight. However, every time they put on the new prescription, they appear to be able to see better; but in reality, their vision is getting worse. The new stronger prescriptions every few years allow them to see for a while until they become so blind that they can't see to find their glasses. My parents used to warn me as a child not to play with glasses. They said that they would make me go blind. Suppression and palliation only makes the patient unaware of the progressive pathological deterioration until the damage has become so great that it is impossible to ever regain sound health.

Our system allows us to examine nature and not accept that which is taught to us from those so-called 'experts.' We have the ability to know what is true and lasting. Our system allows us to take responsibility for our own health. We will not follow some celebrity advertising the next miracle drug. We will not follow some 'important person,' right or wrong. Neither will we follow the popular thing of our time just because it is the easy way out. We must become active in our approach to health.

You may wonder why you haven't been exposed to this truth a lot sooner; and why isn't it in the media; why aren't people singing about it; why aren't movies made about this way to heal all of human's health issues. Well, imagine all of the medical doctors practicing medicine today; there are thousands of hospitals, clinics, and private practices; there are several huge chemical industries making drugs and vaccines; there are thousands of wholesale and retail drug companies employing pharmacists and clerks; there are more nurses than doctors – CNA's, LPN's, RN's and all the other letters of the alphabet; technicians and others who depend on the drug trade for their livelihood. You even have those companies who manufacture bottles, pill boxes, cartons and plastics. You have the newspapers, magazines, radio and television, that receive millions, if not billions, for advertising their products. This means that the drug industry, directly or indirectly, accounts for income that runs into the billions of dollars a year in our country alone. Now, you see why there is a hush-hush on this information. Even those who know don't want to mess up their livelihoods.

My objective is not to stay on the medical profession, but to educate you on true ways of health without the medicine man. However, it seems necessary at times to expose the truth by exposing the lie. If the lie is exposed, then the truth is left standing. The medical profession thinks that we are quacks for saying that the body heals itself; however, many of them has had scrapes and bruises that healed up without the use of anything; and many of them has had broken bones that medicine could not mend back together. The power of the body is the healer in all healings. The body grows and develops itself. If it grows and develops itself, then it also has the ability to heal itself.

However the medical profession might label us, we care less and will continue exposing the truth about the healing ability of the body and their(the curing profession) destructive modes of 'curing.' They can continue to believe what they have been taught in their schools of training. We are appealing to those people who don't make money from the drug trade. They will give ear to this truth, seeing that they do not have a vested interest in the trade.

Our system is a self-care system. It is a system of mind-body care that is free from the poison of drugs or herbal remedies. We do not speak in the Latin or Greek language in educating those health seekers back to health. Our language is clear and easy to understand.

The medical system means to cure consist of about all of the destructive things known to chemist. The chemist has analyzed every substance, both inorganic(lifeless) and organic(with life), of nature. He has created combinations as varied and numberless as the leaves of the forest. Not a mineral or a vegetable poison, however deadly or dangerous, but has been added to the pantry of the medical men to be used to 'cure' man's dis-ease. The poison of insects, of spiders, of snakes, as well as the excretions of animals has been added to the pharmacy and medical man's shelves. Even with all of this searching and using of poisonous stuff in search of a cure, dis-ease has increased; they have become more violent and dangerous. Today we

22

see, with the liberal use of antibiotics, that dis-eases are not yielding to the drugs that the doctors use to treat with them. They are claiming that there is some 'superbug' now. They are admitting that the new strands of viruses are stronger than the antibiotics that they have.

They use a poison(medicine) to poison the germs inside of the body. The use of medicine to kill germs or viruses inside of you is like spraying to kill roaches in your house with insect poisoning spray with the window and doors shut while doing deep breathing exercises. To kill something you must poison it. To kill germs, you must poison them. If they are inside of you, the medical mentality is to swallow poison to kill them.

In breaking the word antibiotic into its two root words, we get anti and biotic. Anti is defined as to mean against, biotic is to mean life. When the two definitions are put together, we get the phrase against life. Our medical profession is fighting dis-ease with a substance that is against life. We are living organisms as well as the germs and viruses. Will not this substance that is against life be against us as well? How can a poison be a way of health? Is it true that a sick person can become less sick by taking a poison that would sicken, even kill them if they were to take it in a state of health?

There was a big fuss about a tea diet that would help its drinkers lose five pounds in five days. People were spending three hundred to a thousand dollars to join and sell the tea. This tea was producing huge dividends for some people and for others the promise of huge incomes. It was difficult to tell these people that this was one very expensive laxative.

23

It only promised five pounds in five days. Most people have many pounds of fecal matter clogged up in their bowels due to overuse or abuse. This tea(laxative) forced the bowels to act on the poisons within the contents of the tea by forcing it out. The fecal matter in the bowels was not as serious as a threat as the poisons contained in the tea. Since the threat in the tea was high, the body acts, even while it was still tired, to rid the body of this toxic substance. So happens, when the bowels voided the toxins, it voided all of its contents including the fecal matter. The bowel was the actor, but the tea got all the praise when the user stepped on the scale and was five pounds lighter. This caused them to buy a second time, but no weight was lost. Why not? Because there was no fecal matter left to expel. Also, every action the body does require the exact amount of rest to replenish its energy reserve to function properly. This means that the more the bowels act and get tired, the more they will require rest to work properly. This type of treatment will force a long rest to be required. A long rest of the bowels is named chronic constipation.

This tea(laxative) forced the sluggish bowels to act as any other bowel action producing drug does. This did nothing for the toxins in the blood and tissues. It did nothing for the accumulated fat in the body. It was only a laxative or poison that irritated the system and bowels to produce bowel action. Might I conclude by saying its praise was short-lived.

See, even the alternative medicine profession is false and misleading. How can you cure the body of its dis-eases with herbs or supplements if the body cures itself? The body is a self-curing organism. It needs no help except that cause is removed and then we follow the ten steps in the preservation or restoration of health, such as: internal and external cleanliness, pure water, adequate sunlight, fresh air, ideal diet suitable for humans, rest and relaxation with adequate sleep, normal temperatures, regular exercise and regular mobility, emotional balance with control of the passions, and nurturing relationships with freedom from violence.

The natural ways of health is ideal for all those beings that have life. Medicine and herbs are not normal or natural. Medicine, or herbs, is not ideal for well individuals to use; but air, water, sun, rest normal temperatures, etc., are all ideal for the well and the sick. The well will stay well as long as they obey the ten ways of health, and the sick will become well as long as they obey the ten ways of health. The reason why the sick is sick is because they have not been obeying those natural ways that I have been mentioning. They are needed for the baby, teenager, adult and elderly woman and man no matter their culture or creed. No one is exempted from these ten ways.

These ten ways of health have been the only way to health since mankind first appeared on earth. If a drug seem to have the power to heal someone, The medical profession would all come together at their conferences and meetings to discuss the possible curative virtues of the drug, but none of them come together when hearing the recovery of the sick using our system to discuss the possible need to stop the medication and start the education of cleanliness, fresh air, pure water, adequate sun, rest and relaxation, ideal diet, normal temperatures, nurturing relationships and the

25

other ways of health that I keep repeating over and over again.

The world hear the praise of some miracle drug or herb everyday, but it never hear about the health restoring ability of the Hygienic System which has helped all those who applied it to their lives. Matter of fact, the hospital is one of the most unhygienic places to be; because there is no sun, fresh air, quietness for rest, or ideal food. But this is where the sick is brought to restore health to their bodies. Take a healthy person and void them of cleanliness, fresh air, pure water, ideal food, sunlight, normal temperatures, rest and relaxation, regular exercise and mobility, or nurturing relationships with freedom from violence and see how long they stay healthy.

Disease: Not The Enemy

It is necessary for you to know that dis-ease is not the enemy it has long been said to be. Instead, it is a remedial process in which the body activates to free itself of the accumulated toxins, to repair some type of damage to the cells and tissue, or a handicap to adapt to continual abuse. When you understand that the living organism is a self-healing organism, you will understand that the caretaker of the sick can only be of value by helping the sick to obey the wholesome conditions and means that produce health.

Health comes from healthy living. Dis-ease comes from unhealthy living. Dis-ease manifests itself by the body to bring the body back to health. The body is always trying to heal itself. Even when you get a scrap on the skin, it bleeds, forms a scab, and heals. The scab protects the wound until the tissues are repaired. Once the tissues are repaired, the scab falls off. Did you or the doctor have any control over that remarkable biological process of healing? No! Healing is a process only accomplished by the body itself.

Dis-ease is not a thing to be removed, expelled, subdued, broken up, cured or killed. It is nothing more than a process or action of the body. Dis-ease is a remedial action that should be left alone to finish the work it was designed to do – which is to bring back a state of balance and health to the body.

If we translate the Latin word acute, we get the English word sharp. This means that an acute dis-ease is a sharp illness. A sharp illness is one that is brought on fast or all of a sudden. The acute crisis is one that is short in duration. The symptoms are commonly severe and there is fever, but the dis-ease does not last long. Examples of acute dis-eases are pneumonia, typhoid fever, meningitis, smallpox, measles, scarlet fever, flu, common cold, etc.

Let's look at diarrhea as an acute action of the body that is sharp, severe and short in duration, but is designed to free the digestive tract of unwanted and non usable material or waste. This is a needed action to free the body of decomposing material; that if not removed, will poison the vital domain. This is an acute crisis to bring about a means to an end of a life threatening situation. Normal elimination is not severe as when the bowel causes a diarrhea to hurry along poisonous materials through the digestive tract to be voided from the body. Once the offending material is removed, the acute crisis(diarrhea) stops and regular bowel movement resumes. Should the diarrhea be stopped or fought with medical or herbal drugs? What would become of the offending material that is threatening the integrity of the organism? Notice that when the body produces a diarrhea to cleanse the bowels it is called a dis-ease, but when a herbal or medical laxative causes a diarrhea in a constipated individual it is called a cure.

Let's look at inflammation as an action of the body; is it not a general response to toxins or injury within or on the surface of the body? If we were to slam our hands in the door or burn it in a fire, the area exposed to the damage

28

becomes inflamed. No other part of the body is inflamed except the damaged area. This means that the inflammation is local to the one area where the damage took place.

Why does inflammation come to damaged areas? Is it not to repair the damage areas? After the slam of the door injure the hand, it becomes swollen, red and with pain. Pain is the language that the body uses to let you know that something is wrong or damaged and that we should not use that part of the body until repair of it has been completed. The area is red and swollen due to the extra blood being sent to the damaged area. The extra blood is being sent to the area because it has the materials needed within it to repair the damaged area. Should we take some form of medication to stop this inflammation process of healing? Would the area be repaired without the materials it needs for repair brought by the extra blood? When the inflammation is left to do its job, the job is completed fast and safe. When the inflammation is stopped or slowed by anti-inflammatory medications, we see that the damage area heals slow or not at all. Most times that area becomes the area where our chronic problem will be. The inflammatory process is a process to bring about healing to a damaged area.

The irritation of toxins irritates the cells within and on the surface of the body. The toxins in the digestive tract irritates and inflame the tract; that's why the diarrhea is initiated by the body to free itself from the toxins. The inflammation is liken to home depot, Lowe's, or some other form of home improvement center that delivers materials to the worksite for construction and repair. A house with broken windows would require few trucks and materials and is finished rather quickly, but a house that has been burn down to the ground requires much more material and the work may go on for a longer period of time. The inflammation is the process of the body to transport material and manage a construction site.

So, acute dis-ease seems to be a means or mode that the body creates to rid itself of toxins or to repair itself from damage. This means that an acute dis-ease is not your enemy but a friend to help preserve life. However, the cause of toxins of damage must be stopped or removed. No one can expect to rebuild a house before putting out the fire that is causing the damage to it. First, put out the fire; then, start to build that which has been damaged. This is common knowledge to carpenters in rebuilding damaged houses, but the medical profession is lacking this common understanding in rebuilding health. In other words, the cause of dis-ease must be removed; and after doing so, there is power within the organism to do the rest towards health.

It is also necessary for you to know what chronic means. A chronic dis-ease is a long lasting dis-ease that usually continues for the remainder of the individual's life. Although the individual may experience acute symptoms in chronic dis-ease, the symptoms are not as severe as those in acute dis-eases. Examples of chronic dis-eases are chronic arthritis, gastric ulcers, most nervous dis-eases, etc.

30

As we have learned that the acute crisis seems to come on suddenly or just 'flare up,' the chronic crisis has developed over time due to continued accumulation of toxins, continued damaged, and suppression of the acute crises that were trying to heal the body. Instead of the body ridding itself of toxins or repairing itself, it tolerates the toxins and attempts to repair damage at an extremely reduced pace.

Dis-ease is merely the crisis of repair, elimination, or adaptation. When the crisis of repair or elimination is hindered by continued cause and/or suppression of drug medications, it develops into a chronic state. This is when the cells, tissues, organs, and whole systems lose their functions and integrity ending in a long term misery that usually ends in death. The acute dis-ease differs because it usually ends with the sufferer returning to a healthy state, provided that the cause is removed. Acute being short in duration battles with toxins and repair work, whereas chronic being ongoing repair work and toleration of toxins.

Forcing the sick tired organs of the sick body into action with stimulants and other drugs is as intelligent as forcing a tired sick horse into greater effort with a whip across his backside. In doing so, he may die from exhaustion and the damage from the whip. You should not whip a tired sick horse to work when tired, and neither can you stimulate a sick tired organ into action in the human body. You will quickly whip and stimulate them to death. Literally!

From the first cough, sneeze, fever, etc., to the last stage of cancer, the body has been working to repair itself from damage and free itself from toxins that have been created

31

within due to metabolism and those from without that are due to personal habits and environmental conditions. Usually the elimination organs detox the body efficiently to not allow toxins to accumulate; but when these organs become fatigue from continued work and no rest or the whipping of medicine, They eventually falter in their jobs of detoxification. This means that instead of the toxins being removed from the blood, tissues and cells, they tend to accumulate irritating the areas they accumulate in. The body, in all its wisdom, searches for alternative routes in which to remove the toxins from the blood, tissues and cells. These routes are what we call acute dis-eases or crises of elimination. When the body has become fatigue from crisis after crisis, it then loses the ability and energy to initiate these alternate routes to ridding itself of the toxins that has been accumulated. The only thing left then is to store, or tolerate, the toxins in the body. This is where the dis-ease becomes chronic. If at anytime the sufferer would cease to produce toxins, or bring them in from without, faster than the body can expel them, the acute dis-eases will never lead to chronic dis-eases.

A lot of people will read this book hoping to learn of some magic remedy or concoction in which to take to cure them of all of their troubles. If not with hopes of cure, they wish to suppress their pain and dis-comforts that they may enjoy again the habits that caused their illnesses. The smoker wants his coughing to stop so that he may enjoy another pull from his tobacco. The diabetic wants their sugar levels reading normal on the meter so that they may resume eating those foods and in the manner that produced their elevated levels. None of them wish to learn how to

32

bring about true health or how to maintain it for life being free from suffering. They only wish to wash, or appear to be clean, that they may go back and play in the mud again. Do they not think that they will get dirty again?

By now, the reader should have a better understanding of the cause of dis-ease and its nature. The nature of dis-ease is how it evolves from a simple 'cold' to irreversible degeneration(cancer.) We no longer have to think that the cause of dis-ease is based on the belief that the invasion of evil spirits or germs have taken over the body and is causing it to act abnormal. We don't have to think that God or some other divine entity Inflicted pain upon us from the heavens.

Old age doesn't mean that we have to suffer from dis-ease that is said to be normal as we age. If this is not true, although it is, why then do we see those dis-eases of old age in our youth more now than ever before? Our youth are dying from dis-eases that were only seen in those who were well advanced in age. We should understand that we bring dis-ease upon our self and our offspring. We do it by disobeying the ten ways of health that we've been discussing so far, such as: cleanliness, fresh air, pure water, adequate sunlight, ideal foods, rest and relaxation, regular exercise and mobility, normal temperatures, emotional balance with control of the passions, and nurturing relationships with freedom from violence.

The Whole Body Is Alive

If you haven't realized yet, humans are very complex beings; and is perfect and marvelous when in obedience with nature. Even when we become disobedient, the body has the ability to survive for a long time; and has the ability to return to obedience and become marvelous again. Obedience to the ten ways of health is all that the organism needs to enjoy perfect health. Disobedience to the ten ways will, in time or quickly in some instances, destroy the organism causing early death. Only a couple of the ten ways can be violated for extended times without causing immediate death. Violation of water and rest may bring on death faster than violation of sun exposure or cleanliness. However, violation of air can bring speedy death faster than the other ways, but this don't have to be always the case.

Being so complex, we posses a mind that gives us the capability to have a higher standard of health than the lower animals. Why don't wild animals need hospitals, doctors, medicine, herbs, supplements, etc.? Are they smarter than us? Were they created to resist germs and viruses and dis-eases that we suffer from? Or could it be that they don't have the habits that we have? And how come the animals that live with humans and follow our ways suffer from our dis-eases? This must mean that the personal habits and conditions that humans live in will produce dis-ease in any living thing that is subjected to the same habits and conditions.

The body is a miraculous thing. It has the ability to arrange as parts of its own structure elements from its surrounding to maintain its vital integrity. This means that it takes from nature what it needs to build and repair itself. To replace old worn out cells they must get elements from outside of the body to make new cells. The body even has the ability to reject and refuse anything brought into its domain that it can not use or threatens its integrity. In plants or animals, from a simple microbe to the most complex organism, assimilation and growth, refusal and rejection are in constant action within. It does so that it can develop and maintain its existence, and to preserve itself from dangerous material.

The body has trillions of cells that make up organs, tissues and complete systems. The organs, tissues and systems make up the organism. Every cell is alive and active in the process to provide the whole with an end product called life. Each cell contributes its efforts in the survival of the organism. There is unity in the body. The digestive system feeds the entire body and not just itself. The respiratory system breathes for the entire body and not just for itself. The cardiovascular system transport nutrients to the cells and remove their waste for the entire body. Every cell and organ has a specific job to keep the organism in operation. All cells, tissues and systems are in cahoots for the survival of the whole organism. None can decide to work alone, and none can decide that it doesn't need the help of the others. It's not like the head can tell the feet that it has no need of them. How then will the head have mobility to get around? The same is true with the internal environment in the body. The digestive tract cannot work

35

without the oxygen provided by the respiratory system, and neither can the lungs breathe without the nutrients for energy provided by the digestive tract when it digests food. The organism is liken to a car assembly line; all stations must do their part to produce a whole car that operates smoothly.

When the cells are always defending themselves from poison or repairing themselves from damage, they can never reflect perfection. Scar tissue is not a beautiful sight to see. Beauty is the reflection of wholeness and of health. Imagine coming home to a dirty house everyday. If you have to scrub toilets, wash dishes, sweep and mop, dust and make up beds, when will you ever have time to paint, hang up pictures, and other larger projects? If the body is always correcting damages we cause to the body and eliminating toxins we keep introducing to the body by our personal habits, when will it have time to beautify us?

Health means to have a sound body and mind. Positive emotions and control of the passions, along with physical integrity, is what we call health. Doctors of today slap a clean bill of health on individuals as long as they are not lying on their sick bed. Most times these people are one foot out of the grave, and some are waste deep. I've had people tell me that they are healthy while they are on three different types of medicine. They say that their health is improved by their medication since the instruments that test them says that they are in the normal range as long as they are taking the medicine. This would make sense if a patient brain dead on a life support machine could say that they were really alive. The health is controlled by magic in both cases. Take the brain dead person off of life support and they will have no action: take the others off of their medicines and their diseases will pain them as it did in the beginning. Take the support away from them both and you will see the true condition of the body. Believe me when I say that it wouldn't be considered healthy.

Partial beauty, fading beauty, decaying beauty is partial, fading, and decaying health. If we are conscious of our stomach, bowels, heart, lungs or any other part of our body, there is something wrong. Health would be uninterrupted if the ten ways of health are obeyed. Breathing fresh air is effortless, but breathing in a dust storm is difficult.

Our habits are so opposite for health in almost every important respect. We eat, drink, smoke, play, work, rest, marry, bear children, go wherever we wish, wherever our appetites and passions leads us all without reference to the laws that govern our bodies. The body needs fresh air, but we stay cooped up in our houses and buildings. The body needs only pure water, but we drink sodas, teas, coffee, alcohols, and other unnatural drinks. We disobey all that is worthy to have perfect health and then wonder why we are sick and start blaming it on the devil or little germs. Some even believe that they may have an evil curse on them. They go to the religious man to pray the curse off of them, and the others go to the doctor to poison the virus out of them or cut out the damage done by the virus.

Dis-ease does not appear overnight. It was long in the making. It takes years of disobedience in most cases to become chronic. It takes some smokers years of smoking to develop lung disorders. It takes the glutton years of wrong

37

eating to develop gastric disorders. It takes years for the drug abuser to suffer the effects from their abuse of the drugs. The alcoholic doesn't get liver cancer from the first sip of alcohol.

Our system is a true way to lasting health. A true way to health is the foundation to our teachings; and everything that is built upon it is true to science and true to the laws of our being. It is a way to keep our bodies at the highest levels of health. It is also a way of living that will allow those that are suffering from dis-ease to regain vibrant health. This way of living is for the well and sick, young and old, male or female, light-skinned or dark-skinned, short or tall if they are to be healthy. Health comes from obeying the ten ways of health. Dis-ease is the result of accidental, ignorant or willful violation of the ten ways of health.

Our system studies and looks at the living nature around us and its needs to preserve and maintain life. We do not look at the dead substances in this nature to preserve and maintain life. We must obey nature rules if we are to have health. Her ways are simple and free to all that wish to have vibrant health. Nature only demands that you breathe fresh air eat the ideal foods that were designed for the human body, rest and relax, maintain freedom from violence, etc. If these things are good for the beast of the forest, why not would it be good for man?

Our system has us to look at the cause of dis-ease in our personal habits and environmental conditions. We look at the type of food that we are eating, the air we are breathing, the type of water that we are drinking, the activities that we are performing or not performing, the

38

amount of rest that we are getting, the temperatures that we are exposing ourselves to, how clean we are keeping ourselves and our surroundings, the level of peace in our lives, the amount of hope and cheer we have, our relationships and their ability to provide us with love, etc.

Our system teaches us of the evil of excesses of any kind. It teaches us how fear, worry, anger, anxiety, internal conflicts, the wrongs of poisons of any kind, deficiencies, and the evils of over sexing.

By now you should see that I have been educating you on two systems or two ways that we look for health, but only one way leads to true health while the other leads too weakness, chronic issues and premature death. One system believes that the personal habits and environmental conditions of the sick sufferer must be changed if they wish to get well. The other system believes that if the right medicine, herb, supplement, or treatment is used, the sufferer may become 'normal again', or at least able to return back to their destructive habits. One believes that a tired organ needs rest in order to regain function and to preserve it. The other system believes that a tired organ needs to be stimulated(forced) into action; but when fatal exhaustion results, they feel that it can then be cut out and replaced with one from a dead person that doesn't need it anymore. You should be able to see how the two systems differ.

The nutrition teachers of today know nothing about the functions of the digestive tract; else they would not be recommending those food groups they call basic to be eaten at the same time. They would not be encouraging the meat

39

and bread diet that they provide for our children's lunch meal. These doctors that go along with these nutrition 'experts' unexpert teachings of eating and drinking will give no attention to those combinations as being a reason to cause a dis-ease. Instead of asking the patient what they are eating and drinking, they will search for germs and viruses. They will ignore coffee, tobacco, alcohol, candy, cookies, chips, excesses, late hours, sexual over-indulgences, over-stimulation of the emotions, etc., and will make the sick person believe that they are sick because of some uncertain, or mysterious, something called disease that has overtaken their bodies and now need to be destroyed. This is where the drugging or cutting begins.

Our system teaches us that we are the builders of our own dis-eases, and it offers us the ten ways of health. The ten ways of health doesn't mean that there are ten different routes that the sick sufferer can choose from to regain health; it is to mean that all ten ways must be practiced and followed altogether to regain vibrant health. We could not think that health can come from food alone, but we must obey all of the ten. What good is eating the healthiest of food, while poisoning ourselves with alcohol, teas, and coffee? What good is drinking the cleanest water while in an area that has us breathing toxic air? What good is eating, drinking, and breathing right if we neglect rest and sleep? We must apply all ten ways to health to reach soundness of mind and body. None of the ten ways can be neglected, and neither can any of them be over-indulged in. Moderation should be the rule in these wholesome things. There should be no moderation or any usage of the unwholesome things.

We are asking you to be moderate in the things that the body require and need for growth, development and reproduction. Be moderate in your eating, drinking, exposure to sun, sex, etc. Drinking too much of the purest water can kill you or cause a dis-ease. Maybe ten or so years prior to this writing, a radio show had a contest to see how much water a person could drink and how quick. They had this one lady who quickly gulped down a gallon or more. Soon after, she collapsed and died. Water lingers in the stomach for about ten to fifteen minutes. After the stomach, it goes into the blood. Water dilutes and thins the blood. The more water taken into the blood, the thinner the blood will be. Blood is the transport system to feed and remove waste from all of the cells of the body; and as such, it is made up of all the materials needed for the cells survival. When water dilutes the blood to the point that materials such as oxygen and food nutrients are thinned out, the cells will die from starvation. This means that the blood has been water-logged. Even the cells become water-logged from the excess. There can be no physical life without the cells alive.

If the cells of the lungs die, what will supply the body with the oxygen it needs from the air? If the cells of the heart die, how will the blood flow? The body is a unit and must be treated as such. I don't mean treated by medicinal or herbal means, but rather looked at as a whole. Abuse to one area will cause the entire organism to suffer. Damage livers will usually always put added pressure on the kidneys; and then they will soon fail also. As there is unity in the human race, since we are subject to the same air, water, sun, earth, etc., there is unity in our bodies. All of the cells,

41

organs, tissues and systems are bound together in one organism working together to provide us with life.

The Cause and Nature of Dis-ease

The medical mentality is neck deep in the germ theory. They believe all, or most of all, of our sufferings are caused from some tiny, minute, only seen under a microscope organism. This theory was brought into practice originally by Louis Pasteur. They believe that viruses invade the body and set up home, all the while causing our sufferings.

How can a person appear 'perfectly healthy' one day and then hocus-pocusly unexplainably stricken with a dreaded dis-ease virtually overnight? They believe that touching some infected doorknob or the shake of a coughed in hand will infect the healthy person causing them to suffer illness. They have labeled over ten thousand categorized dis-eases with their own special names. They even say that each dis-ease has its own cause or causes. They are unaware that there is but only one cause of dis-ease manifested in different ways and locations. The one cause to all dis-ease is TOXEMIA. You will understand that statement better as you continue to read. They spend billions of dollars and countless hours researching the causes of dis-ease without ever looking at the behavior of the sick individual. They are on a wild goose chase for some germ.

The medical profession looks at the nature of dis-ease as being some kind of inevitable thing we must all experience as we age, so they fight it as something that must be destroyed. They feel that we were born to go downhill in our health. They do not take in account for the years of wrong habits and conditions the sick person has went

43

through. Instead, they 'treat' with drugs, herbs, therapy and/or surgery with hopes of making the sick get well. They sometimes explain to you that you will just have to learn to live with dis-ease, especially if their treatments cannot help suppress the pain any longer. It is a new fad for them to tell us to claim our dis-ease and be happy, and to not allow it to stop us from enjoying our life. The religious man tells you to not worry because you will receive a new body at resurrection day.

The thing that the drugging professions and the cure mongers don't realize, and those who do know won't tell you, is that the body heals itself through a biological process. As the fetus is formed in the womb by this process into a complete healthy organism, the same process is needed for the maintenance of the organism. The body is the only healer in all healings. Drugs don't heal anything, but instead they hinder the healing process by suppression. Drugs only allow us to palliate the symptoms of our dis-ease. A simple scratch will heal with or without a bandage. Broken bones may need to be set, but they cannot be mended by any drugs or doctors. They have to be mended by the body itself. This proves that the body heals itself. Look at the woman who had a C-section for birth of her child; the wound is only stitched back together, but time is required for the skin to reconnect to each other. Medicine doesn't have this power. This is power within the body. This is what we mean when we say the body heals itself by a biological process of healing. What heals and mends the bones? What stitches and mends the internal and external wounds? The body is the healer and actor in all healings.

44

When an acute crises of healing begin in an individual, it is to relieve the body of a toxic internal environment or the repair of damage to restore sound integrity of the organism. The body almost always acts in its best interest. The acute symptoms are just the body's way of detoxifying or repairing the body. Sneezing is freeing the nasal of dust, debris and mucus accumulation. The cough is freeing the lungs of debris and mucus accumulation in the lungs and bronchial tube. The diarrhea is freeing the digestive tract of putrid and decomposed waste. The skin eruptions are a route to release toxins through the skin. These are all crisis situations.

We all would leave through the front door to our house if we wished to go somewhere, but we would jump out the window if the door was blocked and a fire(crisis situation) broke out. If the door and windows are blocked, we would search for other alternate routes; maybe we would try busting through a wall. Whichever route the body uses to free itself of the accumulated toxins is considered the safest and fastest route by the brain. To suppress the cough, sneeze, diarrhea, and any of the acute crises, will only force the body to seek other alternative routes that are really dis-comfortable to use. Continued suppression(blocking) will eventually cause the toxins to become trapped causing our chronic problems. Blocking or suppressing an acute dis-ease is like blocking all of your escape routes to free you from a burning building.

We should look at drugs as being a short term effect to a problem that causes longer problems in the future. I usually call drugs differed excuses or bail bonds awaiting trial. You

45

may use a drug to suppress its symptoms, but you are only putting it off for a later date; but, by then, you have accumulated more toxins. This is the same as accumulating more debt with more differed payments and committing more crimes with other bonds. A day will come where you will have to pay all the debt at once or stand trial for all of your crimes.

Taking energy drinks, and not acquiring rest and sleep, does not give you energy; instead, it stimulates the body to use the energy that was stored in the body. This causes the body energy reserves to become more depleted. The short-term effect of the energy drink was one of 'renewed?' energy, but the after effect of the energy drink is a long crash where we would have to sleep even longer to replenish the energy reserve back to a safe level. If energy drinks gave us energy, why would we ever need to rest or sleep? Any time fatigue came to us we should be able to pop the top and down an energy drink or take another pill. The short term effect may occasion more energy, but the long term effect is longer sleep to recuperate. This even explains the acute suffering; the first effect is pain and uncomfortable symptoms, but its long term effect is improved health. The diarrhea is a short term effect that ejects waste material forcefully out of the bowels, but the long-term effect is a healthy digestive tract.

The nature of dis-ease starts with a term we call ENERVATION. Enervation is a depletion of vitality or functioning power. Every cell in the body runs on energy. When those cells are lacking in energy or vital power, they do not function properly. If the power company cuts your power off, your lights will not work. If the lights are not on, how will you see? If the cells are not functioning, they will falter in their job functions. Each cell has a function it must perform to do its part to keep the organism alive an active. We have organs inside the body that does the cleaning and housework to keep a clean inner environment. These organs are the bowels, kidneys, skin, liver, lungs, etc. They are in charge of neutralizing and eliminating toxins away from the cells. If the cells don't remain clean, they prematurely die. The dead cells then become a source of toxins in the body that will have to be neutralized and eliminated.

Why do the eliminating organs falter in their job of house cleaning? They do so because of abuse or overuse. They only get rest when the internal environment is nice and tidy. They refuse to rest while work needs to be done. Any time the level of toxins accumulates higher than the body can tolerate, they have to get it down and keep it in safe levels. Look at the alcoholic that drinks a lot of alcohol. The alcohol is poison coming in from without. This poison must be neutralized and eliminated before it causes death to the body. This means that the liver must work fast and overtime to neutralize the toxins for safe elimination through the kidneys. This means that the kidneys have to work overtime eliminating the neutralized toxins sent from the liver. If not neutralized, the toxins will damage the kidneys. When the liver can't do their job due to fatigue or damage, the kidneys soon follows and becomes dis-eased too.

We can even look at high blood pressure treatment. The doctor gives the sufferer diuretics(water pill) to force fluid off of the body. What organ filters fluid out of the body? The

47

kidneys! That's why we see the sufferer start with high blood pressure and end up with kidney failure. The elimination organs do not rest until they have accomplished their job. Their job is to keep the blood clean. All of the eliminating organs pull waste from the blood to be voided from the body. Only when they have work so much overtime, with no rest, do they become fatigue or enervated.

Now, when these organs become fatigue from the continued use or abuse of them, the toxins begin to accumulate in the blood. This is the condition I spoke of earlier called TOXEMIA. Toxemia is poison or toxic blood. Tox is to mean poison and emia is to mean blood. This blood is the vital fluid that travels to every part of the organism supplying its nutritive material and removing its waste. When this vital fluid becomes toxic, it cannot pick up more waste from the cells or take new materials to the cells. The blood is just a saturated pool of waste. This blood is still in contact with every cell. The toxins within it irritate the cells when they come in contact with them. What cause the filthy blood? Fatigue or damaged elimination organs. What caused the fatigue of the elimination organs? Abuse or overuse by failing to follow and obey the ten ways of health. You will understand this more as we continue.

After the toxins begin to irritate the cells of the body, it causes them to become inflamed. This inflammation causes you to actually feel pain now. The cells or organs that suffer the most are the ones that have been abused the most by our lifestyle and environmental habits; and, at times, a weakness inherited from the parents. This is a weakness in the DNA. This is considered the generational curse. Our bad habits don't just make us suffer, but it also causes defects in our offspring's DNA. Dis-ease will usually manifest itself in the weakest link - the weakest link being the abused, overused or inherited weakness.

The body can find an alternate route to rid itself of its toxic environment by ulceration. The body will release toxins by any means necessary. The skin eruptions will allow the toxins to be eliminated through the skin. Toxins may come through the lungs and expelled by sneezing, mucus dripping from the nose, coughing phlegm forcefully from the throat. There are many ways to expel toxins out of the body; however, this is an acute crisis that we usually hinder by using drugs or herbs. The body mustards up its energy to fight of these poisons, but we resort to drugs to suppress the body's effort of cleansing that we may not have the temporary dis-comfort of the cleansing.

If we want to live long without dis-ease, we have to avoid TOXEMIA. We should not let our blood become toxic. We accomplish this by keeping the body with high energy levels. We keep high energy to function properly by following the ten ways of health. If we don't, our tissues will become hard from the constant irritation of the toxins. This happens when we continually suppress the alternative routes and keep the building up of toxins by our habits. Remember that I called these alternative routes acute crises of elimination. When the crisis is suppressed, the toxins are left in the body causing death to the cells at a fast rate. This toleration is known as a chronic dis-ease because the condition has gone from a quick cleansing process to a long standing toleration of the toxins. Most times the body will put the toxins in out of the way areas such as: joints, arteries, fatty tissues, tumors, and cysts. The chronic problem is due to the toleration of toxins that have been suppressed and palliated. Where the toxins escape the body is seen as an acute crisis of elimination; and where the toxins are stored, and the damage they cause, is seen as a chronic dis-ease.

The nature of dis-ease went as follow: Low energy that made the organs of elimination falter in their job of elimination. This caused a poison blood condition called toxemia. The poisons in the blood irritate the cells to the point that they become inflamed. The body ulcerates to free the toxins from the body. Suppression of the abnormal route of freeing toxins from the body will cause the body to tolerate the poisons by storing them in the body. The cells that are located where these poisons are stored will become hard and die. Dead cells lead to a dead organism. This is the nature of ALL dis-eases if not from the result of direct physical damage to organs, but the nature will still be in this sequence only second to the direct physical trauma.

Our explanation of dis-ease is more logical than any of the other boogieman concepts that are provided by the cure mongers who wish to empty your pockets and bank accounts for their magic potions, pills and gadgets. Our explanation is understood by all that wish to understand truth and doesn't have an interest in the stock of the curing business. Our system doesn't offer any kind of panacea to health; we only educate the sufferer into a healthy way of living that will cause health to be the rule. We do not have to worry about searching for the itty bitty teeny weeny germ, virus, or bacteria as the cause of our health problems such as dis-ease and premature death. Instead, we can look at our lifestyle habits and environmental conditions to see if they will produce disease or health.

It is necessary to understand that whatever will destroy health cannot restore it; for what makes the strong weak, will not, cannot and never will cure or make the sick weak individual strong. And what will aid in restoring a sick person to health will not and never did make a well person sick, not even a little bit. Tobacco smoke may cause the healthy lung to become dis-eased, but it can never cause a dis-eased lung to become healthy from its use. Can you make a drunken man sober by pouring more alcohol down his throat? Giving alcohol to a sober and drunk man will cause one to become drunk and the other to stay drunk. Poison is poison to the well and to the sick person. The living organism, well or sick, is the same organism that requires, if to remain well, and requires, if to regain health when sick, the ten ways of health.

All drugs are poisonous including the herbal remedies. All of them cause dis-ease to some degree, because each one produces another dis-ease. Laxatives causes a diarrhea, diuretics cause kidney failure. All drugs work to tear down the integrity and wisdom of the body. The conditions for health are always the same. The same elements that produce health are also needed to restore health when we have lost it. The sick and well person requires cleanliness, pure water, adequate sunlight, fresh air, ideal food, normal temperatures, regular exercise and movement, rest and sleep, emotional balance and nurturing relationships. The

51

sick requires it to regain health, and the well requires it to maintain their health. We should know by now that sickness is the result of not following the ten ways of health. At any time, the sick follows the ten ways, they will regain health. At any time, the well neglects the ten ways of health, they will suffer dis-ease. The ten ways of health are required for the growth, development, and reproduction of the organism. This means that they are required for health and life. So, when they are required but are lacking, dis-ease will result. When dis-ease is the result, applying the ten ways of health to the body will cause health to result.

Imagine a world with no oxygen, inability to rest and sleep, sun, water, cleanliness, fruits and vegetables or plant life, stable temperature, ability of movement, control of our minds, people to relate with. This is a hell to live in. A heaven would consist of cleanliness, pure water, sun, fresh air, fruits and vegetable and other plants, normal stable temperatures, ability of movement, ability to get rest and sleep, control of our minds, and people in which to relate to and love. Devils are said to live in hell, and Angels are said to live in heaven, not to sound religious, but Angels are always shown as beautiful creatures while devils are always pictured as ugly creepy suffering creatures. Dis-ease is a hell of a situation; whereas, health is a heaven state of existence.

We tend to create our own hellish situations or produce our own heaven. The ten ways of health, for the most part, is a personal care of self. You, alone, are in charge of your cleanliness. You can supply your body with the cleanest air and water. You make the choice to rest and sleep and obey the other ways of health. This seems to mean that disobedience to these ten ways is actually suicidal, because we are doing it to ourselves. The needs of the sick person are not extraordinary, exotic or rare. They do not require the great skill of a doctor's administration of drugs and/or therapy. The multiple degree 'experts' are not needed to safely and efficiently restore the sick back to health. Simple knowledge and application of the ten ways of health can keep the well healthy and restore the sick back to health.

Some have asked the question, "Where are your experiments?" They are asking for experiments for our ten ways. Do they require experiments to prove that we cannot live without air? Do they really need us to prove that fresh air is superior to toxic air? Should we provide more studies on the benefits of rest and sleep? Why should we resort to the laboratory to show that toxic relationships can be ruinous? Nature is our laboratory of life; and however we heed to her laws and principles, will determine if we suffer from dis-ease or have vibrant health. It is up to us to decide between the two by our actions.

Understanding Vital Energy

When understanding vital energy, we must get you to understand that we are talking about functioning power that is generated in the cells (mainly in the brain) that are used to allow functions and processes that are vital to our existence of life to continue. This means that the cells generate their own energy at a low-grade when supplied with air, water, sunlight, food, rest and adequate drainage. When the cells are healthy, they produce high energy. When they are dis-eased, they produce little to no energy. This causes the body to run on back up reserves of the physical, mental, and emotional bodies. Depletion of all energies causes a fatal exhaustion. This means that the organism has no power to operate.

Some have called vital energy an inheritance allotted every cell according to its integrity. If the cell is healthy, it gets a greater amount of inheritance. If the cell is unhealthy, energy can only be accepted in small amounts. This means that the cell that is not allowed to grow, develop and reproduce, is one that will produce little to no energy depending on how damaged and worn out the cell is. High energy is only generated from fresh healthy cells.

The body is the builder and vital energy is the energy of the builder. Air, water, food, sun, is the materials in which to build the house. The other ways of health keep the builder energy level high. The builder requires energy and right materials to build the best house in the least amount of time. The more energy and proper materials the builder have the greater and quicker will the house be built. The best materials in balance produce a mansion or castle.

When we maintain high energy levels, it allows us to have more functioning power for vital processes so that we may have healthier and vibrant lives. The body even stores unused energy in a reserve fund to be used later. AN ENERGY BANK! There's the secret to keep high energy to keep the organs functioning properly. Just as I spoke of reserve energy being used suggests that it must first be able to be saved.

Vital energy is a constant low-grade of electricity created within the cells. When the cells are healthy, they produce a lot of energy; even to the point of excess. This excess is placed in a reserve in a special reserve bank that allows you to make withdrawals and deposits. Rest and sleep are huge deposits to this fund. Fasting is another lottery check to be placed in the reserve fund. Keeping our banks full will mean that we will never suffer from low functioning power. When the reserve bank is depleted, the electricity is cut off from the body. Low functioning power is the cause for the one and only dis-ease named TOXEMIA. Toxemia starts the acute crisis and the decent into dis-ease has begun.

The way of health is simple and plain to understand and do. The first thing is to stop the waste gates of vital energy. Where are you wasting energy should be your first question when acute symptoms present themselves. We only have to look two places – personal habits and environmental conditions. Those personal habits and environmental conditions that are not in line with the ten ways of health

55

need to be corrected immediately. You generate energy by getting rest and sleep, and save energy with the other ways of health. High energy is the ultimate protection against toxemia. Toxemia is the only dis-ease. If you protect yourself from the only dis-ease that manifest many different symptoms in various parts of the body, you will have uninterrupted health.

PART TWO

THE TEN WAYS OF HEALTH EXPLAINED

1.Cleanliness

Cleanliness is one of the ways of health that I have been mentioning. This means to keep external and internal purity. If the external is not clean, then it will be filthy and attract the appropriate parasites that eat away filth; but at the same time, their waste that they leave behind is as, or more, toxic than the filth on the outside of the body. If the internal is not clean, then we develop the condition we call toxemia. Remember, toxemia is the cause of all dis-ease. If filth is in the body, it irritates the cells to the point of hardening and death. The organs that suffer first are the organs that are being abused, overused, and are unclean with the filth of toxic build-up.

External cleanliness means keeping the body, hair, nails and teeth washed and clean. This has to be done everyday, especially in an active person or works around filth. A person who is not so active can be moderate in their washing practices. We suggest that upon rising from sleep, a wipe off would be sufficient. Before we retire to go to sleep, we should take a shower for the duration of approximately five minutes. The shower should be five minutes and the drying off should be ten to fifteen minutes in duration. The drying off is longer due to the need to gently rub the skin. This will allow you to remove the dead cells from the skin as you dry off. The water should be room temperature, and no kind of soap should be used unless you work a very extremely dirty job. Shampoos, conditioners and all other forms of chemical or non-chemical cleansers should not be used on the skin or hair. A quick in and out shower and dry off is the Hygienic way to maintain external cleanliness without wasting the body's energy. As I said, the only time soaps should be used is if the individual has a job similar to a mechanic with grease build-up. However, seldom does the average person have the kind of job that requires that kind of scrubbing with solvents and soaps.

The temperature of the water means a lot about if you are going to use or save your energy to take a shower. Showering, or bathing, with hot water will cause the body to use its energy towards cooling down so that the enzymes are not destroyed within it. It takes energy to produce sweat and activation of the cooling system of the body. If the water is cold, or freezing, the body will use its energy to warm itself up to preserve its integrity so that we don't freeze to death. This is a waste of the vital energies by forcing cold water on the body. Be it hot or cold, wrong temperatures cause a waste of energy to maintain the body with a normal temperature to sustain life. More of this will be spoke of in the section on normal temperatures.

External cleanliness also means the environment that you live in should be clean as well. You cannot expect to live in a pig pin and expect to be healthy. Neither should your surroundings resemble the pig pin. No standing piles of trash or objects should be in your living areas. Decaying trash and mildewing clothes is toxic to your environment. Many objects collect more dust which contaminates your breathing air.

Internal cleanliness means keeping the bodily fluids and tissues pure and free of toxic build-up by avoiding low functioning power. Functioning power is vital power. By maintain high levels of vital power, toxins will not accumulate in the blood causing toxemia or unclean blood. When the blood stay fresh and clean and free from toxins the body tissues will stay soft and pure; and allow the organism to radiate with vibrant health.

Keeping the external and internal is a way of health. Health comes from healthy living. Unclean internal and external environments are both ways to produce dis-ease. This means that if the internal or external environment causes the body to use up its energy dealing with filthiness, it will quickly reach a point of enervation. Enervation means that the vital energies are low and unable to provide the body with the energy required for it to function correctly. So, to avoid the needless waste of energy, keep the external and internal clean.

2.Adequate Sunlight

A weed may grow in the shade, but the finer fruits are found in the sun. A tadpole, if deprived of sunlight, instead of progressing into a respectable frog, will remain a tadpole or degenerate into some unsightly horror. Not only is the sun rays beneficial to the vegetables and other organisms, but it is also absolutely necessary for human life and existence. If we wish to have health, we can no longer deny ourselves adequate exposure to the sun. We need the sun rays for its warmth and its other elements.

The sun should be taken directly on the skin. This is called sun-bathing. The direct rays touching the skin have a host of benefits towards health. The sun rays help the body to absorb and digest calcium. The body produces vitamin D in the cutaneous tissues(tissues beneath the skin) when the sun interacts with the bare skin. It has also been connected in some kind of way to the reproduction of red blood cells. This means that exposure to the sun will help in avoiding anemia. The list of benefits of the sun are numerous to list here; however, I listed a few that you may understand the value of acquiring adequate sun so that you may have health and avoid all those issues that arise from the voidance of it or the lack thereof.

The sun should also be taken through the eyes. Taking sun through the eyes is called sun-gazing. Sun-gazing is ideal for maintain or acquiring optimal eyesight. It also allows for better rest and sleep at the day's end. The pineal gland sits behind the eyes and one of its functions is to regulate our sleep cycle with its production of a hormone termed melatonin. When melatonin is released, we fall to sleep fast and effortlessly. When melatonin is not released, we are wide awake unable to fall asleep. The hormone is released in darkness and is suspended in light. This means that when you are in total darkness, melatonin is being released and you will be compelled to go to sleep; and when you are exposed to sun or light, the production of melatonin comes to a screeching halt. This is why you tend to become sleepy and tired while in a dark room; but when someone opens the curtain, sleep disappears.

This is why it is important to get adequate sunlight throughout the day so that you can get proper sleep to restore energy levels back up from what was used during the day. We will talk about rest real shortly and its benefits; but for now, sun exposure is a way of health that I encourage you to religiously receive as it helps the body assimilate, digest, and produce nutrients needed for health. It also helps the pineal gland rest so that it is able to produce high doses of melatonin to help us fall asleep to restore our energy levels back up. We cannot lay in the dark all day; else we would use up all of the melatonin before night, and we won't be able to go soundly to sleep. If it has been being produced all day, the pineal gland will suffer fatigue. Remember, dis-ease come from overuse or abuse. This means that adequate sunlight should be incorporated into the health seekers daily routine.

I suggest that twenty to thirty minutes of sun on the front and twenty to thirty minutes on the back of the body. We should do the sunbathing before ten in the morning or after three in the afternoon. When sun-gazing in the beginning, the eyes should be closed - allowing the sun to penetrate through the closed lids of the eyes. This can continue for about a week or two; then after, the eyes can be open to look directly at the sun. Don't overdo the sunbathing or sun-gazing, but keep it in moderation. So, if you don't want to be blind as a bat that never gets sun, and you want strong bones with good muscle tone, expose yourself to the sun rays without the hats, sunglasses, sun tan lotions or the over clothing.

3. Pure Air

We cannot eat or drink oxygen. We can only breathe oxygen from the air around us. The air is the source from which we extract our oxygen from. If we are deprived of air for only a few minutes, we will die. This is why fresh air is a way of health, and toxic filthy air is a way of dis-ease and premature death.

We have a pair of lungs with air sac cells designed to exchange carbon dioxide for oxygen on an ongoing basis. It is said that 125 barrels of blood flows throw the lungs for this exchange daily. The lungs are where the impurities are brought from the cells to be eliminated out through them as we exhale. The lungs are also where the blood absorbs the fresh supply of oxygen to take to all of the cells to naturally stimulate their various functions. The fresher the air we breathe, the healthier we will be.

When the air we breathe is toxic and filled with poisons, the unhealthier we will be due to the lack of normal stimulation that the cells need to perform their normal functions. When the cells are unable to function, this is dis-ease. Starving the cells of oxygen will cause them to harden and die. The cells create the organs and systems that create the organism. If the cells die, the organs will die; and then the organism. The cells are the thread of the organism, and without them there is no life or functioning.

When we think of toxic air, we think of outside air that is contaminated from a manufacturing plant or a neighbor's bonfire. However, there are toxic chemicals that are in our homes and at our jobs that are under our own control. Most of us spend the majority of our time indoors breathing toxic air. With our doors and windows shut, we inhale scented items, cleansing products, pesticides, gas from the stove, hair sprays, deodorants, air fresheners, etc. These things pollute the air we breathe. Air fresheners only cover up a smell by overpowering the olfactory senses with a stronger violent scent. The same filth is in the air, but now it has an added odor poisoning the breathing air. Where is the oxygen in air fresheners? Candles uses up the oxygen in your area to keep the flame burning. Void a fire from oxygen and it goes out. Our homes are energy efficient; meaning that no air can come in or go out. This means that we are in a sealed box.

Seal tight in our homes! This means that we can only breathe the air that is in our sealed box. Where will new oxygen come from when we have breathed all the oxygen available in the box? As we breathe in the oxygen, we exhale carbon dioxide. This means that our internal air is changing rapidly from oxygen to high levels of carbon dioxide. With all the other toxic chemicals in the house, it resembles us living in the garage with the doors down while the car is running. Some of us even smoke in our sealed boxes. We continually breathe over and over again the toxins produced from our personal habits and those lingering in our environment. Our homes need to be ventilated and allowed to let fresh air circulate at all times.

Oxygen is necessary for the bodily processes that sustain our lives. The air we breathe furnishes this oxygen. When our air is mixed with other toxins and poisons, we have less oxygen available to breathe. We know that toxins are not the way of health. We should know that the fresher our air is, the fewer toxins will be breathed in. Fresh air vitalizes the cells. This means it will help save and produce energy for the body. The more energy, the better the body functions. The better the body functions, the less chance toxins will accumulate in the blood producing toxemia. No toxemia, no dis-ease.

Therefore, we need to breathe the freshest air. The freshest air is always found outside in the open. We should exercise outside so that we can breathe deep and get the benefits of the fresh air. We need to ventilate all our areas of life. We can keep clean and get adequate sun; but if we don't receive the oxygen our body needs, it will lead to dis-ease and premature death. Let's not hide from the open air.

4.Pure Water

All of the chemical-vital processes or changes that take place in the body require the presence of water. When the body is lacking, or becomes dehydrated, disturbances of the operations become known very fast. We can see that the tissue of the body that contains the least water, such as the bone or nails, has little vital inheritance. Tissues that are merely for support or protection are low in water, but the active tissues are high in water. We see this in muscles, glands, nerves, and the brain.

Water has no taste, smell or color; that's if it is pure water. In examining the many forms of water that is available to us, only water that has been filtered and vapor distilled would constitute as H^2O(water.) Anything added to this chemical formula H^2O makes it something other than water. Minerals added to the water alter its chemical formula. This means that it is no longer pure; but instead, it is contaminated with materials other than two parts hydrogen and one-part oxygen. In chemistry, water is two parts hydrogen and one-part oxygen; and to add anything to this mixture changes its formula. When you change the formula, you get another mixture that cannot be used by the body. Anything added causes the water to become toxic and impure. Impure means that it has been altered and is no longer fit for what it was designed for.

When we look at gold, we tend to want the purest because we know that it is of the greatest value. Now, if we add other metals to dilute its purity, it becomes less in value. In fact, the more it has of the other metals added to it, the more worthless it becomes. The same is true with water. The purest we acquire our water, the more of value our body will benefit from it. The more impurities added to the water, the more toxic and worthless will it be to the body. Instead of using the water, it will use up its energy expelling it out or trying to clean it for use. Both are a waste of the vital power needlessly since it will be used in cleanup work. This means that no energy is wasted when we supply our body with fresh pure water. This means that more energy is saved and used to keep the body cleansed of toxins form within and not from those brought in from without. One drink leads to health, and all others are a sip closer to dis-ease.

Water is very important to the body; so, it would be wise to use the best that you can for your body. This body belongs to you. The best water is water that has been filtered and vapor distilled. The body is around seventy-two percent water, in which the average person holds forty-four quarts in their body. Water is continually being lost from the body when we sweat, urinate, breathe, and through bowel action. There are three ways by which we can replace this lost; through the fluids we drink, through the foods we eat, and through the oxidation process where hydrogen forms as a byproduct of digestion and combines with the oxygen we inhale.

We should acquire the purest water by drinking distilled water. We should eat the foods that are highly water-sufficient, such as fruits and vegetables. This is important if one wants to have health. Health comes from cleanliness; which means that our water must be clean as well. The agriculture farmers would be laughed at if they poured sodas, unnatural juices, kool-aids, sports drinks, coffee, tea or any other watery toxins on their crops. When the harvest season come, he will have nothing to harvest. In fact, it would cause the death to their business and cause a famine in the land. Why, then, do we think that we can nourish our bodies with these types of concoctions and grow, develop, and reproduce? As the plant needs the cleanliest water, so does humans require such cleanliness. Pure distilled water is the water that should be used when sick or well.

The smart water company boasts about their product being distilled water, but they made the mistake of adding minerals for taste. They cleaned the water and then added dirt back to it. Let us not get caught up on the health frenzy that is depleting the people out of their pockets and their health. When thirst presents itself, satisfy it with pure distilled water.

5.Rest and Sleep

The way to health is to avoid enervation. Enervation is when our functioning power has reached a very low level. When the body becomes low in energy, it doesn't function normally or at all. This is a cause of dis-ease. The way to keep all of the cells functioning, and not in a state of dis-ease, is to supply them with the energy they require by avoiding enervation. This brings us to rest and sleep. Sleep is the only way to generate energy at a rapid rate and resting is next in line. Without rest and sleep, the body quickly runs out of energy and organs and systems starts shutting down due to low functioning power. This means that they are no longer able to function efficiently.

Systems and organs require rest. The cells require rest. The muscles require rest. None of them can continue long without rest before reaching a point of exhaustion. The stomach is a muscle that requires rest like all other muscles. The muscles of the jaw, small intestines and large intestines that produce the peristaltic motion needed to move material through them, and other muscles require rest as well. When we continually eat, we are constantly forcing these muscles to work. Not allowing them to rest makes them less capable of performing efficiently in their duties. A tired horse is not efficient as a rested horse.

If low energy is the cause of toxemia, and toxemia is the root to all dis-ease, then we should avoid allowing our energy levels to reach a low level. This is accomplished by

70

getting proper sleep and rest. How do we get proper rest? Relax and fast often. How do we get proper sleep? Get adequate sun during the day and be active; then find a quiet dark place in the evening and lay flat with lite bedding. Do not have night lights, televisions or radios on. This will assure that you get the proper sleep you need to generate maximum functioning power.

Think of it this way: your cell phone is fully charged; you use it to make calls, text, take pictures, and search the web. Doing one of those activities drain the battery slow, but doing them all at the same time depletes the battery rapidly. You can charge the phone while those things are still going on, but it won't restore the energy as fast as if the phone was turned off. The phone will also charge faster when none of its applications are being used. Our body saves energy when it is inactive at a rapid rate. This means that sleep is the fastest way to restore the energy reserves of the individual who is suffering from enervation. Sleep is the only way to recharge the body's battery at the fastest rate; because when we are active, we are depleting the energy faster than we can produce it and accumulate it.

The vital energy has been said to be our inheritance. Every living particle is endowed with this life force called vital energy or nerve energy. It is a constant supply of energy generated in the cells for their usage. The energy is created faster in youthful healthy cells and not so fast in old worn out hard cells. That's why the wounds of the young heal quicker than those of the elderly. This is high energy we are witnessing in these children as they run around like they have ants in their pants. This energy usually makes the elderly tired by watching the youth. This is low energy that we are witnessing in the elderly.

Your cells produce energy just like the cells of solar panels. The older the solar panel cells, and the more worn out and damaged that they are, the less energy they will produce. The solar panel cells will have to be replaced by a workman. The great thing about the body is that they reproduce their own cells. They replace themselves according to the nutrients they have in which to build themselves. The cells use water, air, food, sun and etc. in which to build it. The body is the builder and the water, air, food, sun, etc. is the materials it uses to build. When the builder is fatigued, nothing can be built. When the builder is full of vitality and functioning power, the building is built fast and to perfection. But the builder can only build according to the materials on hand. That's why we have been teaching you that the requirements for health are the materials of building. Once you get the rest you need, the body then has the functioning to rebuild itself to perfection according to its ability. Then we should supply the body with the other ways of health and watch a mansion or castle being built. Proper rest and sleep is mandatory for good health.

6. The Ideal Diet

You can go to any fuel station today and pull up to the fueling pumps to three different types of fuel. They are considered as three grades of fuel known usually as premium, silver, and regular. The different grades provide either inferior or superior fuel to our vehicles. The cleaner fuel protects and allows the car to run smooth for the longest time. The inferior fuel has little protection and causes us breakdown prematurely. No one likes for their car to breakdown.

We can go to the grocery store and food places and see the various kinds of food available for us to eat to fuel our bodies to produce energy. We have vegetables, meats, starches, and process and refined foods. Vegetables are superior to the other foods and meats and process refined foods being inferior. I must say that fruits are the premium food for the body. The fruits and vegetables, eaten in their whole and uncooked state, provide the body with the organic materials it needs to repair its structures. Fruits and vegetables are the best means by which to keep the cells healthy and vibrant. Meats and unnatural foods build the body with unhealthy material causing low-grade structures to be formed. This means that the unhealthy structures will be unable to produce high levels of functioning power. This means that the body will operate sluggishly from the bad fuel we're using to fuel it with. We should know that our bodies will operate vibrantly when we feed them the premium foods that promote health and longevity.

The ideal diet is fresh wholesome uncooked fruits, vegetables, nuts and seeds. These should be eaten in a combination that allows proper digestion in the stomach. The stomach has a ph factor. Certain foods are acidic while others are alkaline. This means that when acidic foods are eaten, alkaline foods should be left alone. Acidic and alkaline foods should not be eaten at the same time. If they are, the stomach mixture will not be mixed correctly to breakdown the food eaten. Acidic foods require an acid medium in the stomach to be present to aid in the breaking down of the food. Alkaline foods require an alkaline medium to be present in the stomach to aid in the breaking down of the food. When these two types of food are eaten at the same time, both mediums are poured into the stomach. This means that the medium is neither acid nor alkaline, but neutral. This means that the acidic food cannot be broken down due to the wrong digestive mixture, and the alkaline food cannot be broken down due to this same wrong mixture. This will cause none of the food to be in a mixture that is able to break them down. So, this means that nothing will get digested.

If the food we eat doesn't get digested because of our wrong combinations, it cannot fuel the cells. In fact, the food will linger in the digestive tract longer than it should. While sitting in the stomach longer than they are suppose too, they start the decomposing process. Instead of digesting and fueling the body, it rots turning into toxins that poison the body. Remember, toxins is the cause to all of our dis-eases. As this is the case, the body has to use unnecessary energy to eliminate the toxins produced from our wrong combinations. This needless use of energy robs the body of its reserves leading us faster to the state of enervation.

The ideal diet should also be eaten when in an emotional balance. This means that your emotions should always be in check. You should not eat when in fear, worry, or even when excited. It takes energy to digest food and it takes energy to deal with our emotions. Religions have always suggested that we pray and get our minds right before eating. This practice calms the emotions and sets the tone for the meal. Fear causes the stomach to knot up making it unable to churn the food to digest it. Many animals, such as the snake, will regurgitate their meal in order to fight or flight if there's a threat with fear.

Notice how a holiday meal makes everyone sleepy or tired and fatigued after eating. There is not much anyone wants to do after those large crazy combined foods. This is also a time of excitement where friends and family are together having fun. The reason for the sleep is to conserve the energy to digest, or deal, with this conglomerate of material thrown into the system.

We sometimes eat and hurry back to our jobs of laborious activity. This means that, instead of using the energy towards digesting food, the energy is used for work and activities. This means that the food has to wait longer in the digestive tract pending the supply of energy in which to digest the food. While the food is waiting to be digested in the stomach, it is subject to decompose and rot. This is a

75

source of toxins that will poison the system. Most times the body will produce a diarrhea to free the decomposed food out of the system fast and safely. However, this diarrhea uses up a lot of the body's reserve energy. When the body's energy reserve is constantly called on to free up the digestive tract by producing a diarrhea, it soon reaches enervation. When enervation is reached, toxemia begins. When toxemia begins, the dis-ease process is well on its way.

The way of health here is to eat the ideal diet of fresh uncooked fruits, vegetables, nuts and seeds. This diet should be eaten uncooked so that the enzymes of the food are not destroyed by the heat from cooking. It should be eaten in the right state of mind and balance. To eat unnatural, cooked, refined or processed foods under stress, excessive excitement, or just simply eating it period will result in low energy and the formation of toxic materials from the decomposing food when it doesn't get digested. The reason it rots fast is because the stomach is warm, wet and dark. This type of environment favors rapid decomposition. This is why it is ideal to eat foods that are easily digested and combined correctly. The ideal diet is a way of health if we wish to have health.

7.Normal Temperatures

Humans run a temperature between 98 and 99 degrees. This is what the medical science considers to be homeostasis. This means that it is the ideal temperature for the body to conduct its functions and affairs. If this temperature gets low or high, it will stress the body and hinder its activities. All the cells of the body have a job to do in providing us with an end product called LIFE. If the cells are damaged due to the cold or hot temperature, they will cease to provide the body with the prize product we all want for a very long time.

It is a great thing that the internal temperature is regulated by the brain. When we expose ourselves to the extreme cold or heat, our bodies have to use energy to keep warm or cool down. This is energy that could have been used for elimination or repair; but instead, it was used to regulate the body's temperature so that the cells don't freeze or overheat. It has to maintain the 98 or 99 range to be ideal for the body to function properly.

Since the energy is being used for controlling and regulating our temperature from our unnecessary exposure to the cold or heat, the organs of elimination will be lacking in their energy. When the organs of elimination are lacking in their energy, they falter. When they falter, toxins accumulate in the body causing toxemia. Toxemia is the root to all dis-ease.

So, avoiding the waste of energy by having to have the body warm itself from the cold and cool itself from the heat, more energy will be saved for the elimination organs to eliminate the toxins from the body. When the toxins are eliminated fast from the body via high energy elimination organs, this brings growth, development and reproduction to the body. This means that we won't suffer dis-ease since there won't be a toxemia. Toxemia is the root to all dis-eases.

Normal temperatures are a way of health that saves energy to be used by the body for elimination and repair work. Energy not used for personal habits and environmental conditions, is energy used for functioning power. The elimination of toxins is efficient and the repair process is efficient. This is the body function at its highest ability. This is what we consider health.

When we drink cold drinks or hot ones, the stomach is either paralyzed from the cold or weakened and relaxed from the heat. A stomach cannot digest food when it is shocked and paralyzed from the cold; neither can it churn to digest the food when it has been weakened and relaxed from the heat. We all have applied heat to a muscle to relax them, so we know that the same must be true for the stomach muscles.

So, it is important that we only expose ourselves to normal temperatures that do not waste our precious energy or hinder the digestive process. This is a way of health.

8.Regular Exercise and Mobility

Regular exercise and mobility is a way of health by keeping the body fit and strong. The cells are cleansed by movement via the lymphatic system. The lymphatic system is similar to the circulatory system, except it doesn't have an organ that circulates its fluid through the body. Lymph fluid is the fluid that bathes the cells and removes their waste and dumps them into the blood. The only way to move the fluid from the cell to the blood is by movement.

When the blood becomes toxic with waste that is generated from within and without, the lymph has no place in which to dump the cells waste in. If the blood is already toxic, no more toxins can be dump into it. The blood cannot become acidic; so, it will either neutralize the toxins by borrowing from the bones calcium, the nerves potassium and the muscles calcium to make the toxins safe for storage, or ulcerate from the body as an acute crisis of elimination using abnormal routes that are a dis-ease. We say both are the way of dis-ease.

If the body robs from its bones, they break easily; If from the nerves, they become shaky and jittery; If from the muscles, they become weak. These are all symptoms of dis-ease and illnesses. Maintaining the alkaline minerals reserves high in the body will result in healthier cells and organs. This is accomplished by eating alkaline foods such as

79

fruits and vegetables, and avoiding toxic build up in the blood and lymph that cause the body to have to steal from its reserves to neutralize the toxins.

There are three forms of exercises that we should incorporate in our routines: stretching, aerobics, and weightlifting. These three will keep excellent movement that will insure that lymph is moved through the body. When lymph is moved through the body, the cells will remain clean. Clean cells produce high energy and remain youthful longer. Keep movement and high energy levels so that your cells can stay young and vibrant.

9.Emotional Poise

A poised person is said to be a person of grace, balance or control. The poise of the physical body is a man standing in a great posture and balance. The poise of the emotional and mental bodies must be balanced and standing in a great posture to have whole health. If the mental is unbalanced, we have mental disorders(we can also see this in individuals who has had trauma to the brain.) If the emotions are unbalanced, emotional diseases develop(this too can result from trauma to the brain.) When these bodies are not in good standing, we suffer dis-ease. It is a good emotional poise to be calm and gentle in all matters. It is a good mental poise to meditate and think on positive things. These things bring about balance and control in those areas.

Keeping emotional poise is when we stay free of addictions; when we operate in high self-esteem; when we agree to serve a purpose that is deserving of praise and commendation with worthy healthy goals. The way to balance must first purify the mind, body, and emotions. This is whole health when the mind, body and emotions are healthy and balanced.

Emotional health is a very important part of the key to happiness and health. When the emotions are out of balance, the physical and mental body will suffer as well. When you express anger or hate, your muscles tense up and adrenaline flows preparing you for a fight or flight response. This adrenaline is irritating to the cells. It is used to

81

stimulate them into action. Stimulation is irritation. The mental is affected by the emotions with thoughts that eventually cause more of the physical sensations. This cycle of emotions that causes a physical sensation and mental thought continues until all of our vital energy has been used up. This produces a state of enervation. Enervation brings on toxemia.

Imagine the person who suffers from ulcers of the stomach that is due to stress. This person has been eating foods while the stomach was unable to digest the food. This caused irritation from the food. Inflammation followed the irritation; which finally reached a state of ulceration. Stress requires a lot of energy. This means that, when the body is under stress, mental or emotional, food should not be taken. This also means that the energy of the body is being wasted dealing with stress. This will bring on enervation at a rapid rate. When enervation is brought on, toxemia soon follows. Toxemia is the root to all dis-ease. Many of us have lost body functioning during fright, worry, and fear. This means that emotions have the ability to produce physical disorders. So, the way of health is to keep the emotions calm and balanced.

10.Nurturing Relationships

Most of the times when we tell health seekers about the importance of positive relations over negative relations, we are thought to mean only the relations between a male and female: as in a husband and wife relationship. Nurturing relationships are needed in all of the relationships in our lives. The way you relate to mom, dad, sister, brother, job, dog, etc. must be nurturing and positive. Toxic relationships can cause destructive habits, direct danger, or unnecessary emotions that lead to emotional, mental and physical disorders.

The toxic relationship with a dog can be: attacking you physically by biting you; barking all night causing you to get a headache or no sleep; becoming so angry that your muscles tense up. The animal cannot be growling at you keeping you agitated or in fear. These will soon result in physical symptoms. Neither can we have other relationships in our lives that physically attack us, mentally attack us, or emotionally keep us unbalanced. Family, friends, jobs and all other relationships should be healthy and positive. Our dog should lick, instead of biting; have us smiling, fearless and happy, instead of angry, mad, and fearful.

Anything that deserves your relations in this life, are ones that do not attack you physically, mentally or emotionally. You will know because each emotion has an equally balanced mental and physical, be they negative or positive, action at the same time. It doesn't matter which of the two

83

came first but a physical sensation, mental thought and emotional feeling will happen like a domino effect. You think of a dead loved one (the mental thought); you become sad (emotional feeling); your head begins to ache or your stomach begins to feel queasy (physical sensation). You watch a family member get into a bad accident (an event); they might be dead (mental thought); intense sorrow and sadness (emotional feeling); breathing becomes difficult, chest hurts, stomach knots (physical sensation). The concept here is to keep positive people, places, and things in every area of your life. This is a way of health.

Conclusion

We have learned the true cause and nature of disease. We have learned the fallacy in the medical understanding on disease. We have supplied you with the true knowledge and way of health that is superior to all others for the exchange of your present uneducated understanding. We say that it is uneducated because it is founded in the medical mentality. The medical mentality is based on falsehoods and is misleading. We have sufferers that are suffering from diseases from the past and present that have been prolonged and palliated. This has caused them to never look or search for the true ways of health. We do not believe that there is a way to health that doesn't employ the ten ways discussed in these words. Any approach to health that doesn't apply and endorse these ten ways is misleading.

Our ten ways of health is a simple system that can be understood by the elderly and small children alike. It can be understood by the woman as well as he man. It is a system of self care and a science that relates to human nature. Without the ten ways of health disease will be the rule. When we apply cleanliness, fresh air, pure water, adequate sunlight, ideal diet, rest, regular exercise, normal temperatures, emotional balance, and nurturing relationships, health will be the rule. These ways of health should not be abused or over used. So, Natural Hygiene, as our science is called, is the preservation and restoration of health by using unadulterated natural means and influences. Those natural means and influences are what we call, the ten ways of health. Learn these ten ways of health and apply them to the sick and they should get well, provided the recuperative ability of the body hasn't exceeded its ability to do so; and if this is the case, no other healing modality would be of any benefit.